THIS PLANNER

Belongs To:

I'm PREGNANT!

DUE DATE

HOW I FOUND OUT

MY REACTION

WHAT I AM MOST EXCITED ABOUT

WHO I TOLD FIRST

WHAT I WANT YOU TO KNOW

MY BIRTH PLAN *Ideas*

WHO I WANT IN THE DELIVERY ROOM:

TYPE OF BIRTH

- [ ] VAGINAL
- [ ] WATER BIRTH
- [ ] C-SECTION
- [ ] VBAC

THOUGHTS ABOUT BIRTH AND WHAT IS MOST IMPORTANT TO ME

GETTING READY FOR THE BIG DAY: TO DO

NOTES & IDEAS (lighting, music, etc.)

40 Week PREGNANCY *Tracker*

Keep track of how you're feeling every week of your pregnancy.

APPOINTMENT *Tracker*

Keep track of your pre-natal classes and doctor appointments.

DATE	TIME	ADDRESS	PURPOSE

BABY SHOPPING *List*

Start planning for the arrival of your baby by using the shopping list below.

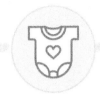

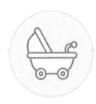

Undershirts	Crib	Bottles
Socks	Bassinet	Bottle Liners
Pajamas	Baby Bath tub	Nursing Bra & Pads
Sweaters	Car Seat	Breast Pump
Onesies	Stroller	Formula
Hats	High Chair	Pacifiers
Bibs	Play Pen	Bottle Brush
Blanket	Baby Swing	Burp Cloths
Diaper Bag	Monitor	Bottle Sanitizer
Mitts	Change Table	Nipples
Diapers	Rocking Chair	Baby Powder
Booties	Night Light	Baby Wipes
Receiving Blankets	Mobile	_____
Crib Sheet	Bouncer	_____
Wash Cloths	Nail Clippers	_____
Towels	Teething Toys	_____
_____	Baby Wipes	_____
_____	Diaper Pail	_____
		_____

Weight PREGNANCY Tracker

Weight Tracker Chart

It's important to keep track of your weight throughout your pregnancy.
Record your weight in the chart below every week, starting at week 4.

WEEKLY WEIGHT TRACKER

4		12		20		28		36
5		13		21		29		37
6		14		22		30		38
7		15		23		31		39
8		16		24		32		40
9		17		25		33		
10		18		26		34		
11		19		27		35		

NOTE According to the American Pregnancy Association, pregnant women should consume up to 300 more calories a day. Further, healthy eating is critical to your baby's development which means you should make sure to maintain a well-balanced diet, high in nutrients and proteins.

HEALTHY FOOD Ideas

VEGETABLES & LOW SUGAR FRUIT	PROTEINS	COMPLEX CARBS	HEALTHY FATS	SUPPLEMENTS
Leafy greens (spinach, etc.)	Organic meat	Beets	Avocado	Vitamin D
Broccoli	Liver	Carrots	Olive Oil	Fish Oil
Cauliflower	Bone Broth	Sweet Potatoes	Coconut Oil	Algae Oil
Cabbage	Beans	Yams	Yogurt	Probiotics
Asparagus	Lentils	Parsnips	Almonds	Ginger Pills
Cucumber	Flax Seed	Turnips	Mixed Nuts	Licorice Root
Mushrooms	Pumpkin Seed	Pumpkin	Soybean	Magnesium
Celery	Chia Seed	Buckwheat	Olives	Krill Oil
Radish	Salmon	Brown Rice	Nut butter	Iron Pills
Grapefruit & Melon	Herring	Squash		
Berries (all kinds)				
Peaches (with skin)				

Tracker PRE-NATAL Visits

Keep track of your pre-natal appointments and include a summary of each visit.

DATE

HOW FAR ALONG?

YOUR WEIGHT

BLOOD PRESSURE

FETAL HEART RATE

DOCTOR

NOTES:

SUMMARY OF APPOINTMENT

NEXT APPOINTMENT.:

DATE

HOW FAR ALONG?

YOUR WEIGHT

BLOOD PRESSURE

FETAL HEART RATE

DOCTOR

NOTES:

SUMMARY OF APPOINTMENT

NEXT APPOINTMENT.:

DATE

HOW FAR ALONG?

YOUR WEIGHT

BLOOD PRESSURE

FETAL HEART RATE

DOCTOR

NOTES:

SUMMARY OF APPOINTMENT

NEXT APPOINTMENT.:

1-13 Weeks

FIRST Trimester

HOW I FELT DURING MY FIRST TRIMESTER

ENERGY

SLEEP

CRAVINGS

MOODS

MY FAVORITE MEMORIES

TO DO LIST: 1st TRIMESTER

SYMPTOMS & CRAVINGS

FIRST TRIMESTER *Photos*

MEMORIES ARE FOREVER

14-27 Weeks

SECOND Trimester

HOW I FELT DURING MY SECOND TRIMESTER

ENERGY

SLEEP

CRAVINGS

MOODS

MY FAVORITE MEMORIES

TO DO LIST: 2nd TRIMESTER

SYMPTOMS & CRAVINGS

SECOND TRIMESTER *Photos*

MEMORIES ARE FOREVER

28-40 Weeks

THIRD Trimester

HOW I FELT DURING MY THIRD TRIMESTER

MY FAVORITE MEMORIES

SYMPTOMS & CRAVINGS

ENERGY

SLEEP

CRAVINGS

MOODS

TO DO LIST: 3rd TRIMESTER

THIRD TRIMESTER *Photos*

MEMORIES ARE FOREVER

MY BABY Shower

BABY SHOWER PHOTOS

GAMES PLAYED

ON THE MENU

HIGHLIGHTS & MEMORIES

MY BABY Shower Gifts

Keep track of your baby shower gifts and send thank you notes

NAME	GIFT	ADDRESS	SENT?

NURSERY *Planner*

COLOR SCHEME IDEAS:

ITEM TO PURCHASE	PRICE	NOTES

FURNITURE IDEAS

DECORATIVE IDEAS

BABY NAME *Ideas*

TOP 3 BOY NAMES

NAME
MEANINGS

TOP 3 GIRL NAMES

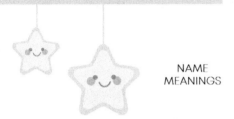

NAME
MEANINGS

BABY NAME RESOURCES (LIST YOUR FAVORITE PARENTING & PREGNANCY WEBSITES):

OTHER BOY NAME POSSIBILITIES	OTHER GIRL NAME POSSIBILITES

HOSPITAL *Checklist*

FOR ME	FOR PARTNER	FOR BABY

PREGNANCY SHOPPING *List*

BABY CLOTHING	SUPPLIES/MEDICATION	FURNITURE/TOYS

FIRST TRIMESTER SHOPPING	SECOND TRIMESTER SHOPPING	THIRD TRIMESTER SHOPPING

FETAL Movement

Starting around week 16, keep track of when you feel your baby move.

WEEK 16	TIME	NOTES
MON		
TUE		
WED		
THU		
FRI		
SAT		
SUN		

WEEK 17	TIME	NOTES
MON		
TUE		
WED		
THU		
FRI		
SAT		
SUN		

WEEK 18	TIME	NOTES
MON		
TUE		
WED		
THU		
FRI		
SAT		
SUN		

WEEK 19	TIME	NOTES
MON		
TUE		
WED		
THU		
FRI		
SAT		
SUN		

WEEK 20	TIME	NOTES
MON		
TUE		
WED		
THU		
FRI		
SAT		
SUN		

WEEK 21	TIME	NOTES
MON		
TUE		
WED		
THU		
FRI		
SAT		
SUN		

WEEK 22	TIME	NOTES
MON		
TUE		
WED		
THU		
FRI		
SAT		
SUN		

WEEK 23	TIME	NOTES
MON		
TUE		
WED		
THU		
FRI		
SAT		
SUN		

WEEK 24	TIME	NOTES
MON		
TUE		
WED		
THU		
FRI		
SAT		
SUN		

Tracker FETAL Movement

WEEK 25	TIME	NOTES
MON		
TUE		
WED		
THU		
FRI		
SAT		
SUN		

WEEK 26	TIME	NOTES
MON		
TUE		
WED		
THU		
FRI		
SAT		
SUN		

WEEK 27	TIME	NOTES
MON		
TUE		
WED		
THU		
FRI		
SAT		
SUN		

WEEK 28	TIME	NOTES
MON		
TUE		
WED		
THU		
FRI		
SAT		
SUN		

WEEK 29	TIME	NOTES
MON		
TUE		
WED		
THU		
FRI		
SAT		
SUN		

WEEK 30	TIME	NOTES
MON		
TUE		
WED		
THU		
FRI		
SAT		
SUN		

WEEK 31	TIME	NOTES
MON		
TUE		
WED		
THU		
FRI		
SAT		
SUN		

WEEK 32	TIME	NOTES
MON		
TUE		
WED		
THU		
FRI		
SAT		
SUN		

WEEK 33	TIME	NOTES
MON		
TUE		
WED		
THU		
FRI		
SAT		
SUN		

Tracker FETAL Movement

WEEK 34	TIME	NOTES
MON		
TUE		
WED		
THU		
FRI		
SAT		
SUN		

WEEK 35	TIME	NOTES
MON		
TUE		
WED		
THU		
FRI		
SAT		
SUN		

WEEK 36	TIME	NOTES
MON		
TUE		
WED		
THU		
FRI		
SAT		
SUN		

WEEK 37	TIME	NOTES
MON		
TUE		
WED		
THU		
FRI		
SAT		
SUN		

WEEK 38	TIME	NOTES
MON		
TUE		
WED		
THU		
FRI		
SAT		
SUN		

WEEK 39	TIME	NOTES
MON		
TUE		
WED		
THU		
FRI		
SAT		
SUN		

WEEK 40	TIME	NOTES
MON		
TUE		
WED		
THU		
FRI		
SAT		
SUN		

NOTES		

Dear Lord PRAYER Time

TODAY'S
DATE

Psalm 90:17

May the favor of the Lord our God rest on us;
establish the work of our hands for us—
yes, establish the work of our hands.

Reflections

_____
_____
_____
_____
_____
_____
_____
_____
_____
_____
_____

Week 4

PREGNANCY Journal

Your baby is the size of a poppy seed!

TOTAL WEIGHT GAIN

BELLY MEASUREMENT

BABY BUMP PHOTO

WEEKLY REFLECTIONS

SYMPTOMS & CRAVINGS

WHAT I WANT TO REMEMBER MOST

I'M MOST EXCITED ABOUT

I'M MOST NERVOUS ABOUT

Dear Baby

Dear Baby

PREGNANCY *Journal*

TODAY'S DATE

WEEKS PREGNANT

HOW I'M FEELING TODAY

What I want you to know

Dear Lord

PRAYER *Time*

TODAY'S
DATE

Philippians **1:6**

Being confident of this very thing, that he who began a good work in you will complete it until the day of Jesus Christ.

Reflections

Week 5

PREGNANCY *Journal*

Your baby is the size of a peppercorn!

TOTAL WEIGHT GAIN

BELLY MEASUREMENT

BABY BUMP PHOTO

WEEKLY REFLECTIONS

SYMPTOMS & CRAVINGS

WHAT I WANT TO REMEMBER MOST

I'M MOST EXCITED ABOUT

I'M MOST NERVOUS ABOUT

Dear Baby

Dear Baby

PREGNANCY *Journal*

TODAY'S DATE

WEEKS PREGNANT

HOW I'M FEELING TODAY

What I want you to know

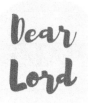

Dear Lord PRAYER Time

TODAY'S
DATE

Psalm 139:14

I will give thanks to you, for I am fearfully and wonderfully made. Your works are wonderful. My soul knows that very well.

Reflections

Week 6

PREGNANCY Journal

Your baby is the size of a sweet pea!

TOTAL WEIGHT GAIN

BELLY MEASUREMENT

BABY BUMP PHOTO

WEEKLY REFLECTIONS

SYMPTOMS & CRAVINGS

WHAT I WANT TO REMEMBER MOST

I'M MOST EXCITED ABOUT

I'M MOST NERVOUS ABOUT

Dear Baby

Dear Baby

PREGNANCY *Journal*

TODAY'S
DATE

WEEKS
PREGNANT

HOW I'M
FEELING TODAY

What I want you to know

Dear Lord

PRAYER Time

TODAY'S DATE

2 Peter 3:18

But grow in the grace and knowledge of our Lord and Savior Jesus Christ. To him be glory both now and forever! Amen.

Reflections

PREGNANCY *Journal*

Your baby is the size of a blueberry!

TOTAL WEIGHT GAIN

BELLY MEASUREMENT

BABY BUMP PHOTO

WEEKLY REFLECTIONS

SYMPTOMS & CRAVINGS

WHAT I WANT TO REMEMBER MOST

I'M MOST EXCITED ABOUT

I'M MOST NERVOUS ABOUT

Dear Baby

Dear Baby

PREGNANCY *Journal*

TODAY'S DATE

WEEKS PREGNANT

HOW I'M FEELING TODAY

What I want you to know

Dear Lord

PRAYER Time

Matthew 8:24-26

Behold, a violent storm came up on the sea, so much that the boat was covered with the waves; but he was asleep. The disciples came to him and woke him up, saying, "Save us, Lord! We are dying!" He said to them, "Why are you fearful, O you of little faith?" Then he got up, rebuked the wind and the sea, and there was a great calm.

Reflections

Week 8

PREGNANCY *Journal*

Your baby is the size of a raspberry!

TOTAL WEIGHT GAIN

BELLY MEASUREMENT

BABY BUMP PHOTO

WEEKLY REFLECTIONS

SYMPTOMS & CRAVINGS

WHAT I WANT TO REMEMBER MOST

I'M MOST EXCITED ABOUT

I'M MOST NERVOUS ABOUT

Dear Baby

PREGNANCY *Journal*

TODAY'S DATE

WEEKS PREGNANT

HOW I'M FEELING TODAY

What I want you to know

TODAY'S
DATE

Luke 1:46-48

"My soul magnifies the Lord. My spirit has rejoiced in God my Savior, for he has looked at the humble state of his servant. For behold, from now on, all generations will call me blessed."

Reflections

PREGNANCY *Journal*

Your baby is the size of a grape!

TOTAL WEIGHT GAIN

BELLY MEASUREMENT

BABY BUMP PHOTO

WEEKLY REFLECTIONS

SYMPTOMS & CRAVINGS

WHAT I WANT TO REMEMBER MOST

I'M MOST EXCITED ABOUT

I'M MOST NERVOUS ABOUT

Dear Baby

Dear Baby

PREGNANCY *Journal*

TODAY'S DATE

WEEKS PREGNANT

HOW I'M FEELING TODAY

What I want you to know

TODAY'S DATE

Isaiah 43:5-7

"Don't be afraid, for I am with you. I will bring your offspring from the east, and gather you from the west. I will tell the north, 'Give them up!' And tell the south, 'Don't hold them back! Bring my sons from far away, and my daughters from the ends of the earth— everyone who is called by my name, and whom I have created for my glory, whom I have formed, yes, whom I have made.'"

Reflections

PREGNANCY *Journal*

Your baby is the size of a prune!

TOTAL WEIGHT GAIN

BELLY MEASUREMENT

BABY BUMP PHOTO

WEEKLY REFLECTIONS

SYMPTOMS & CRAVINGS

WHAT I WANT TO REMEMBER MOST

I'M MOST EXCITED ABOUT

I'M MOST NERVOUS ABOUT

Dear Baby

Dear Baby

PREGNANCY *Journal*

TODAY'S DATE

WEEKS PREGNANT

HOW I'M FEELING TODAY

What I want you to know

Dear Lord

PRAYER Time

♥ ♥ ♥ ♥ ♥ ♥ ♥ ♥ ♥ ♥ ♥ ♥ ♥ ♥ ♥ ♥ ♥ ♥

TODAY'S
DATE

John 14:6

Jesus said to him, "I am the way, and the truth, and the life. No one comes to the Father except through me.

Reflections

PREGNANCY Journal

Your baby is the size of a lime!

TOTAL WEIGHT GAIN

BELLY MEASUREMENT

BABY BUMP PHOTO

WEEKLY REFLECTIONS

SYMPTOMS & CRAVINGS

WHAT I WANT TO REMEMBER MOST

I'M MOST EXCITED ABOUT

I'M MOST NERVOUS ABOUT

Dear Baby

Dear Baby

PREGNANCY *Journal*

TODAY'S DATE

WEEKS PREGNANT

HOW I'M FEELING TODAY

What I want you to know

Dear Lord

PRAYER Time

2 Corinthians 13:14

The grace of the Lord Jesus Christ, God's love, and the fellowship of the Holy Spirit be with you all. Amen.

Reflections

Week 12

PREGNANCY *Journal*

Your baby is the size of a plum!

TOTAL WEIGHT GAIN

BELLY MEASUREMENT

BABY BUMP PHOTO

WEEKLY REFLECTIONS

SYMPTOMS & CRAVINGS

WHAT I WANT TO REMEMBER MOST

I'M MOST EXCITED ABOUT

I'M MOST NERVOUS ABOUT

Dear Baby

ULTRASOUND Scan

ULTRASOUND PHOTO

ULTRASOUND RESULTS

BABY'S LENGTH:

BABY'S WEIGHT:

BPD:

DUE DATE:

Notes

Dear Baby

PREGNANCY *Journal*

TODAY'S DATE

WEEKS PREGNANT

HOW I'M FEELING TODAY

What I want you to know

Dear Lord PRAYER Time

Deuteronomy 7:13

He will love you, bless you, and multiply you. He will also bless the fruit of your body and the fruit of your ground, your grain and your new wine and your oil, the increase of your livestock and the young of your flock, in the land which he swore to your fathers to give you.

Reflections

_____
_____
_____
_____
_____
_____
_____
_____
_____
_____
_____

PREGNANCY *Journal*

Your baby is the size of a peach!

TOTAL WEIGHT GAIN

BELLY MEASUREMENT

BABY BUMP PHOTO

WEEKLY REFLECTIONS

SYMPTOMS & CRAVINGS

WHAT I WANT TO REMEMBER MOST

I'M MOST EXCITED ABOUT

I'M MOST NERVOUS ABOUT

Dear Baby

Dear Baby

PREGNANCY *Journal*

TODAY'S
DATE

WEEKS
PREGNANT

HOW I'M
FEELING TODAY

What I want you to know

Dear Lord PRAYER *Time*

♥ ♥ ♥ ♥ ♥ ♥ ♥ ♥ ♥ ♥ ♥ ♥ ♥ ♥ ♥ ♥ ♥ ♥

TODAY'S
DATE

Luke **1:14**

And you will have joy and gladness, and many will rejoice at his birth.

Reflections

Week 14

PREGNANCY *Journal*

Your baby is the size of a lemon!

TOTAL WEIGHT GAIN

BELLY MEASUREMENT

BABY BUMP PHOTO

WEEKLY REFLECTIONS

SYMPTOMS & CRAVINGS

WHAT I WANT TO REMEMBER MOST

I'M MOST EXCITED ABOUT

I'M MOST NERVOUS ABOUT

Dear Baby

Dear Baby

PREGNANCY *Journal*

TODAY'S DATE

WEEKS PREGNANT

HOW I'M FEELING TODAY

What I want you to know

PRAYER Time

TODAY'S
DATE

Ecclesiastes **11:5**

As you don't know what is the way of the wind, nor how the bones grow in the womb of her who is with child; even so you don't know the work of God who does all.

Reflections

PREGNANCY *Journal*

Your baby is the size of an apple!

TOTAL WEIGHT GAIN

BELLY MEASUREMENT

BABY BUMP PHOTO

WEEKLY REFLECTIONS

SYMPTOMS & CRAVINGS

WHAT I WANT TO REMEMBER MOST

I'M MOST EXCITED ABOUT

I'M MOST NERVOUS ABOUT

Dear Baby

Dear Baby

PREGNANCY *Journal*

TODAY'S DATE

WEEKS PREGNANT

HOW I'M FEELING TODAY

What I want you to know

Dear Lord

PRAYER *Time*

TODAY'S
DATE

Job **31:15**

Didn't he who made me in the womb make him? Didn't one fashion us in the womb?

Reflections

Week 16

PREGNANCY *Journal*

Your baby is the size of an avocado!

TOTAL WEIGHT GAIN

BELLY MEASUREMENT

WEEKLY REFLECTIONS

SYMPTOMS & CRAVINGS

WHAT I WANT TO REMEMBER MOST

I'M MOST EXCITED ABOUT

I'M MOST NERVOUS ABOUT

BABY BUMP PHOTO

Dear Baby

Dear Baby

PREGNANCY *Journal*

TODAY'S DATE

WEEKS PREGNANT

HOW I'M FEELING TODAY

What I want you to know

Dear Lord

PRAYER Time

Luke **1:44-45**

For behold, when the voice of your greeting came into my ears, the baby leaped in my womb for joy! Blessed is she who believed, for there will be a fulfillment of the things which have been spoken to her from the Lord!"

Reflections

_____
_____
_____
_____
_____
_____
_____
_____
_____
_____
_____

PREGNANCY Journal

Your baby is the size of a pear!

TOTAL WEIGHT GAIN

BELLY MEASUREMENT

BABY BUMP PHOTO

WEEKLY REFLECTIONS

SYMPTOMS & CRAVINGS

WHAT I WANT TO REMEMBER MOST

I'M MOST EXCITED ABOUT

I'M MOST NERVOUS ABOUT

Dear Baby

Dear Baby

PREGNANCY *Journal*

TODAY'S DATE

WEEKS PREGNANT

HOW I'M FEELING TODAY

What I want you to know

PRAYER Time

Psalm 139:13

For you formed my inmost being. You knit me together in my mother's womb.

Reflections

PREGNANCY *Journal*

Your baby is the size of a sweet potato!

TOTAL
WEIGHT GAIN

BELLY
MEASUREMENT

BABY BUMP PHOTO

WEEKLY REFLECTIONS

SYMPTOMS & CRAVINGS

WHAT I WANT TO REMEMBER MOST

I'M MOST EXCITED ABOUT

I'M MOST NERVOUS ABOUT

Dear Baby

Dear Baby

PREGNANCY *Journal*

TODAY'S DATE

WEEKS PREGNANT

HOW I'M FEELING TODAY

What I want you to know

TODAY'S
DATE

John 16:21

A woman, when she gives birth, has sorrow because her time has come. But when she has delivered the child, she doesn't remember the anguish any more, for the joy that a human being is born into the world.

Reflections

PREGNANCY *Journal*

Your baby is the size of a mango!

TOTAL WEIGHT GAIN

BELLY MEASUREMENT

BABY BUMP PHOTO

WEEKLY REFLECTIONS

SYMPTOMS & CRAVINGS

WHAT I WANT TO REMEMBER MOST

I'M MOST EXCITED ABOUT

I'M MOST NERVOUS ABOUT

Dear Baby

Dear Baby

PREGNANCY *Journal*

TODAY'S DATE

WEEKS PREGNANT

HOW I'M FEELING TODAY

What I want you to know

Dear Lord

PRAYER *Time*

Jeremiah 1:4-5

Now Yahweh's word came to me, saying, "Before I formed you in the womb, I knew you. Before you were born, I sanctified you. I have appointed you a prophet to the nations."

Reflections

Week 20

PREGNANCY *Journal*

Your baby is the size of a banana!

TOTAL WEIGHT GAIN

BELLY MEASUREMENT

BABY BUMP PHOTO

WEEKLY REFLECTIONS

SYMPTOMS & CRAVINGS

WHAT I WANT TO REMEMBER MOST

I'M MOST EXCITED ABOUT

I'M MOST NERVOUS ABOUT

Dear Baby

PRAYER Time

Dear Lord

Isaiah 43:1-3

But now Yahweh who created you, Jacob, and he who formed you, Israel, says: "Don't be afraid, for I have redeemed you. I have called you by your name. You are mine. When you pass through the waters, I will be with you, and through the rivers, they will not overflow you. When you walk through the fire, you will not be burned, and flame will not scorch you. For I am Yahweh your God, the Holy One of Israel, your Savior.

Reflections

ULTRASOUND Scan

ULTRASOUND PHOTO

ULTRASOUND RESULTS

BABY'S LENGTH:

BABY'S WEIGHT:

BPD:

DUE DATE:

Notes

Dear Baby

PREGNANCY *Journal*

TODAY'S DATE

WEEKS PREGNANT

HOW I'M FEELING TODAY

What I want you to know

PRAYER Time

1 John 5:14-15

This is the boldness which we have toward him, that if we ask anything according to his will, he listens to us. And if we know that he listens to us, whatever we ask, we know that we have the petitions which we have asked of him.

Reflections

PREGNANCY *Journal*

Your baby is the size of a carrot!

TOTAL WEIGHT GAIN

BELLY MEASUREMENT

BABY BUMP PHOTO

WEEKLY REFLECTIONS

SYMPTOMS & CRAVINGS

WHAT I WANT TO REMEMBER MOST

I'M MOST EXCITED ABOUT

I'M MOST NERVOUS ABOUT

Dear Baby

Dear Baby

PREGNANCY *Journal*

TODAY'S
DATE

WEEKS
PREGNANT

HOW I'M
FEELING TODAY

What I want you to know

TODAY'S DATE

Habakkuk 3:18-19

Yet I will rejoice in Yahweh. I will be joyful in the God of my salvation! Yahweh, the Lord, is my strength. He makes my feet like deer's feet, and enables me to go in high places.

Reflections

Week 22

PREGNANCY *Journal*

Your baby is the size of a papaya!

TOTAL WEIGHT GAIN	BELLY MEASUREMENT

WEEKLY REFLECTIONS

SYMPTOMS & CRAVINGS

WHAT I WANT TO REMEMBER MOST

I'M MOST EXCITED ABOUT

I'M MOST NERVOUS ABOUT

BABY BUMP PHOTO

Dear Baby

Dear Baby

PREGNANCY *Journal*

TODAY'S DATE

WEEKS PREGNANT

HOW I'M FEELING TODAY

What I want you to know

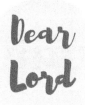

PRAYER *Time*

TODAY'S
DATE

Ephesians **6:10**

Finally, be strong in the Lord, and in the strength of his might.

Reflections

PREGNANCY *Journal*

Your baby is the size of a grapefruit!

TOTAL WEIGHT GAIN

BELLY MEASUREMENT

BABY BUMP PHOTO

WEEKLY REFLECTIONS

SYMPTOMS & CRAVINGS

WHAT I WANT TO REMEMBER MOST

I'M MOST EXCITED ABOUT

I'M MOST NERVOUS ABOUT

Dear Baby

Dear Baby PREGNANCY *Journal*

TODAY'S
DATE

WEEKS
PREGNANT

HOW I'M
FEELING TODAY

What I want you to know

Dear Lord

PRAYER Time

TODAY'S
DATE

Joshua 1:9

"Haven't I commanded you? Be strong and courageous. Don't be afraid. Don't be dismayed, for Yahweh your God is with you wherever you go."

Reflections

PREGNANCY *Journal*

Your baby is the size of a cantaloupe!

TOTAL
WEIGHT GAIN

BELLY
MEASUREMENT

BABY BUMP PHOTO

WEEKLY REFLECTIONS

SYMPTOMS & CRAVINGS

WHAT I WANT TO REMEMBER MOST

Dear Baby

I'M MOST EXCITED ABOUT

I'M MOST NERVOUS ABOUT

Dear Baby

PREGNANCY *Journal*

TODAY'S DATE

WEEKS PREGNANT

HOW I'M FEELING TODAY

What I want you to know

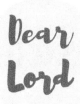

PRAYER Time

TODAY'S DATE

Philippians 4:13

can do all things through Christ, who strengthens me.

Reflections

PREGNANCY *Journal*

Your baby is the size of a cauliflower!

TOTAL WEIGHT GAIN

BELLY MEASUREMENT

BABY BUMP PHOTO

WEEKLY REFLECTIONS

SYMPTOMS & CRAVINGS

WHAT I WANT TO REMEMBER MOST

I'M MOST EXCITED ABOUT

I'M MOST NERVOUS ABOUT

Dear Baby

PREGNANCY *Journal*

TODAY'S DATE

WEEKS PREGNANT

HOW I'M FEELING TODAY

What I want you to know

TODAY'S DATE

Isaiah **40:29-31**

He gives power to the weak. He increases the strength of him who has no might. Even the youths faint and get weary, and the young men utterly fall; but those who wait for Yahweh will renew their strength. They will mount up with wings like eagles. They will run, and not be weary. They will walk, and not faint.

Reflections

Week 26

PREGNANCY *Journal*

Your baby is the size of a head of lettuce!

TOTAL
WEIGHT GAIN

BELLY
MEASUREMENT

BABY BUMP PHOTO

WEEKLY REFLECTIONS

SYMPTOMS & CRAVINGS

WHAT I WANT TO REMEMBER MOST

Dear Baby

I'M MOST EXCITED ABOUT

I'M MOST NERVOUS ABOUT

Dear Baby

PREGNANCY Journal

TODAY'S
DATE

WEEKS
PREGNANT

HOW I'M
FEELING TODAY

What I want you to know

Dear Lord

PRAYER Time

Colossians 1:11-12

Strengthened with all power, according to the might of his glory, for all endurance and perseverance with joy, giving thanks to the Father, who made us fit to be partakers of the inheritance of the saints in light

Reflections

PREGNANCY *Journal*

Your baby is the size of a rutabaga!

TOTAL WEIGHT GAIN

BELLY MEASUREMENT

BABY BUMP PHOTO

WEEKLY REFLECTIONS

SYMPTOMS & CRAVINGS

WHAT I WANT TO REMEMBER MOST

Dear Baby

I'M MOST EXCITED ABOUT

I'M MOST NERVOUS ABOUT

Dear Baby

PREGNANCY *Journal*

TODAY'S DATE

WEEKS PREGNANT

HOW I'M FEELING TODAY

What I want you to know

Dear Lord

PRAYER Time

TODAY'S DATE

Isaiah 40:11

He will feed his flock like a shepherd. He will gather the lambs in his arm, and carry them in his bosom. He will gently lead those who have their young.

Reflections

Week 28

PREGNANCY *Journal*

Your baby is the size of an eggplant!

TOTAL WEIGHT GAIN

BELLY MEASUREMENT

WEEKLY REFLECTIONS

SYMPTOMS & CRAVINGS

WHAT I WANT TO REMEMBER MOST

I'M MOST EXCITED ABOUT

I'M MOST NERVOUS ABOUT

BABY BUMP PHOTO

Dear Baby

Dear Baby

PREGNANCY Journal

TODAY'S DATE

WEEKS PREGNANT

HOW I'M FEELING TODAY

What I want you to know

Dear Lord

PRAYER Time

Psalm 84:11-12

For Yahweh God is a sun and a shield. Yahweh will give grace and glory. He withholds no good thing from those who walk blamelessly. Yahweh of Armies, blessed is the man who trusts in you.

Reflections

Your baby is the size of acorn squash!

TOTAL WEIGHT GAIN

BELLY MEASUREMENT

BABY BUMP PHOTO

WEEKLY REFLECTIONS

SYMPTOMS & CRAVINGS

WHAT I WANT TO REMEMBER MOST

Dear Baby

I'M MOST EXCITED ABOUT

I'M MOST NERVOUS ABOUT

Dear Baby

PREGNANCY Journal

TODAY'S
DATE

WEEKS
PREGNANT

HOW I'M
FEELING TODAY

What I want you to know

Dear Lord

PRAYER Time

TODAY'S DATE

Isaiah 26:3-4

You will keep whoever's mind is steadfast in perfect peace, because he trusts in you. Trust in Yahweh forever; for in Yah, Yahweh, is an everlasting Rock.

Reflections

PREGNANCY *Journal*

Your baby is the size of a cucumber!

TOTAL WEIGHT GAIN

BELLY MEASUREMENT

BABY BUMP PHOTO

WEEKLY REFLECTIONS

SYMPTOMS & CRAVINGS

WHAT I WANT TO REMEMBER MOST

I'M MOST EXCITED ABOUT

I'M MOST NERVOUS ABOUT

Dear Baby

Dear Baby

PREGNANCY *Journal*

TODAY'S DATE

WEEKS PREGNANT

HOW I'M FEELING TODAY

What I want you to know

PRAYER *Time*

TODAY'S DATE

Psalm **55:22**

Cast your burden on Yahweh and he will sustain you. He will never allow the righteous to be moved.

Reflections

PREGNANCY *Journal*

Your baby is the size of a pineapple!

TOTAL WEIGHT GAIN

BELLY MEASUREMENT

BABY BUMP PHOTO

WEEKLY REFLECTIONS

SYMPTOMS & CRAVINGS

WHAT I WANT TO REMEMBER MOST

I'M MOST EXCITED ABOUT

I'M MOST NERVOUS ABOUT

Dear Baby

Dear Baby

PREGNANCY *Journal*

TODAY'S DATE

WEEKS PREGNANT

HOW I'M FEELING TODAY

What I want you to know

Dear Lord

PRAYER Time

TODAY'S DATE

Philippians 4:6-7

In nothing be anxious, but in everything, by prayer and petition with thanksgiving, let your requests be made known to God. And the peace of God, which surpasses all understanding, will guard your hearts and your thoughts in Christ Jesus.

Reflections

PREGNANCY *Journal*

Your baby is the size of a squash!

**TOTAL
WEIGHT GAIN**

**BELLY
MEASUREMENT**

BABY BUMP PHOTO

WEEKLY REFLECTIONS

SYMPTOMS & CRAVINGS

WHAT I WANT TO REMEMBER MOST

Dear Baby

I'M MOST EXCITED ABOUT

I'M MOST NERVOUS ABOUT

Dear Baby

PREGNANCY *Journal*

TODAY'S DATE

WEEKS PREGNANT

HOW I'M FEELING TODAY

What I want you to know

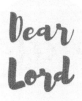

PRAYER Time

Dear Lord

TODAY'S
DATE

Isaiah **41:10**

Don't you be afraid, for I am with you. Don't be dismayed, for I am your God. I will strengthen you. Yes, I will help you. Yes, I will uphold you with the right hand of my righteousness.

Reflections

PREGNANCY *Journal*

Your baby is the size of a durian!

TOTAL WEIGHT GAIN

BELLY MEASUREMENT

BABY BUMP PHOTO

WEEKLY REFLECTIONS

SYMPTOMS & CRAVINGS

WHAT I WANT TO REMEMBER MOST

I'M MOST EXCITED ABOUT

I'M MOST NERVOUS ABOUT

Dear Baby

PREGNANCY *Journal*

TODAY'S DATE

WEEKS PREGNANT

HOW I'M FEELING TODAY

What I want you to know

TODAY'S
DATE

Romans **15:13**

Now may the God of hope fill you with all joy and peace in believing, that you may abound in hope, in the power of the Holy Spirit.

Reflections

PREGNANCY *Journal*

Your baby is the size of a butternut squash!

TOTAL WEIGHT GAIN

BELLY MEASUREMENT

BABY BUMP PHOTO

WEEKLY REFLECTIONS

SYMPTOMS & CRAVINGS

WHAT I WANT TO REMEMBER MOST

I'M MOST EXCITED ABOUT

I'M MOST NERVOUS ABOUT

Dear Baby

PREGNANCY *Journal*

TODAY'S DATE

WEEKS PREGNANT

HOW I'M FEELING TODAY

What I want you to know

PRAYER Time

TODAY'S
DATE

Jeremiah 1:8

Don't be afraid because of them, for I am with you to rescue you," says Yahweh.

Reflections

Your baby is the size of a coconut!

TOTAL WEIGHT GAIN

BELLY MEASUREMENT

BABY BUMP PHOTO

WEEKLY REFLECTIONS

SYMPTOMS & CRAVINGS

WHAT I WANT TO REMEMBER MOST

I'M MOST EXCITED ABOUT

I'M MOST NERVOUS ABOUT

Dear Baby

Dear Baby

PREGNANCY *Journal*

TODAY'S
DATE

WEEKS
PREGNANT

HOW I'M
FEELING TODAY

What I want you to know

Dear Lord

PRAYER Time

Psalm 63:4-8

So I will bless you while I live. I will lift up my hands in your name. My soul shall be satisfied as with the richest food. My mouth shall praise you with joyful lips, when I remember you on my bed, and think about you in the night watches. For you have been my help. I will rejoice in the shadow of your wings. My soul stays close to you. Your right hand holds me up.

Reflections

PREGNANCY Journal

Your baby is the size of a honeydew melon!

TOTAL
WEIGHT GAIN

BELLY
MEASUREMENT

BABY BUMP PHOTO

WEEKLY REFLECTIONS

SYMPTOMS & CRAVINGS

Dear Baby

WHAT I WANT TO REMEMBER MOST

I'M MOST EXCITED ABOUT

I'M MOST NERVOUS ABOUT

Dear Baby

PREGNANCY *Journal*

TODAY'S DATE

WEEKS PREGNANT

HOW I'M FEELING TODAY

What I want you to know

Dear Lord

PRAYER Time

TODAY'S DATE

James 1:17-18

Every good gift and every perfect gift is from above, coming down from the Father of lights, with whom can be no variation, nor turning shadow. Of his own will he gave birth to us by the word of truth, that we should be a kind of first fruits of his creatures.

Reflections

Your baby is the size of a Winter Melon

TOTAL WEIGHT GAIN

BELLY MEASUREMENT

BABY BUMP PHOTO

WEEKLY REFLECTIONS

SYMPTOMS & CRAVINGS

WHAT I WANT TO REMEMBER MOST

I'M MOST EXCITED ABOUT

I'M MOST NERVOUS ABOUT

Dear Baby

Dear Baby

PREGNANCY *Journal*

TODAY'S DATE

WEEKS PREGNANT

HOW I'M FEELING TODAY

What I want you to know

Dear Lord

PRAYER Time

♥♥ ♥♥ ♥♥ ♥ ♥♥ ♥♥ ♥♥ ♥ ♥♥ ♥♥ ♥♥ ♥ ♥♥ ♥♥

TODAY'S
DATE

1 Peter 5:7

Casting all your worries on him, because he cares for you.

Reflections

PREGNANCY *Journal*

Your baby is the size of a pumpkin!

TOTAL
WEIGHT GAIN

BELLY
MEASUREMENT

BABY BUMP PHOTO

WEEKLY REFLECTIONS

SYMPTOMS & CRAVINGS

WHAT I WANT TO REMEMBER MOST

Dear Baby

I'M MOST EXCITED ABOUT

I'M MOST NERVOUS ABOUT

PREGNANCY *Journal*

TODAY'S DATE

WEEKS PREGNANT

HOW I'M FEELING TODAY

What I want you to know

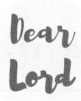

PRAYER *Time*

TODAY'S
DATE

Psalm 127:3

Behold, children are a heritage of Yahweh. The fruit of the womb is his reward.

Reflections

PREGNANCY *Journal*

Your baby is the size of a watermelon!

TOTAL
WEIGHT GAIN

BELLY
MEASUREMENT

BABY BUMP PHOTO

WEEKLY REFLECTIONS

SYMPTOMS & CRAVINGS

WHAT I WANT TO REMEMBER MOST

I'M MOST EXCITED ABOUT

I'M MOST NERVOUS ABOUT

Dear Baby

Dear Baby

PREGNANCY *Journal*

TODAY'S
DATE

WEEKS
PREGNANT

HOW I'M
FEELING TODAY

What I want you to know

PRAYER *Time*

♥♥ ♥♥ ♥♥ ♥♥ ♥♥ ♥♥ ♥♥ ♥♥

TODAY'S
DATE

Psalm 23

Yahweh is my shepherd: I shall lack nothing. He makes me lie down in green pastures. He leads me beside still waters. He restores my soul. He guides me in the paths of righteousness for his name's sake. Even though I walk through the valley of the shadow of death, I will fear no evil, for you are with me. Your rod and your staff, they comfort me.

Reflections

PREGNANCY *Journal*

Your baby is the size of a jack fruit!

TOTAL WEIGHT GAIN

BELLY MEASUREMENT

BABY BUMP PHOTO

WEEKLY REFLECTIONS

SYMPTOMS & CRAVINGS

WHAT I WANT TO REMEMBER MOST

I'M MOST EXCITED ABOUT

I'M MOST NERVOUS ABOUT

Dear Baby

Dear Baby

PREGNANCY *Journal*

TODAY'S DATE

WEEKS PREGNANT

HOW I'M FEELING TODAY

What I want you to know